MATTHEW WHITE

Your Guide to Fitness over 50

Learn The Basics of Getting Fit Over 50 without the Gym

Contents

Introduction

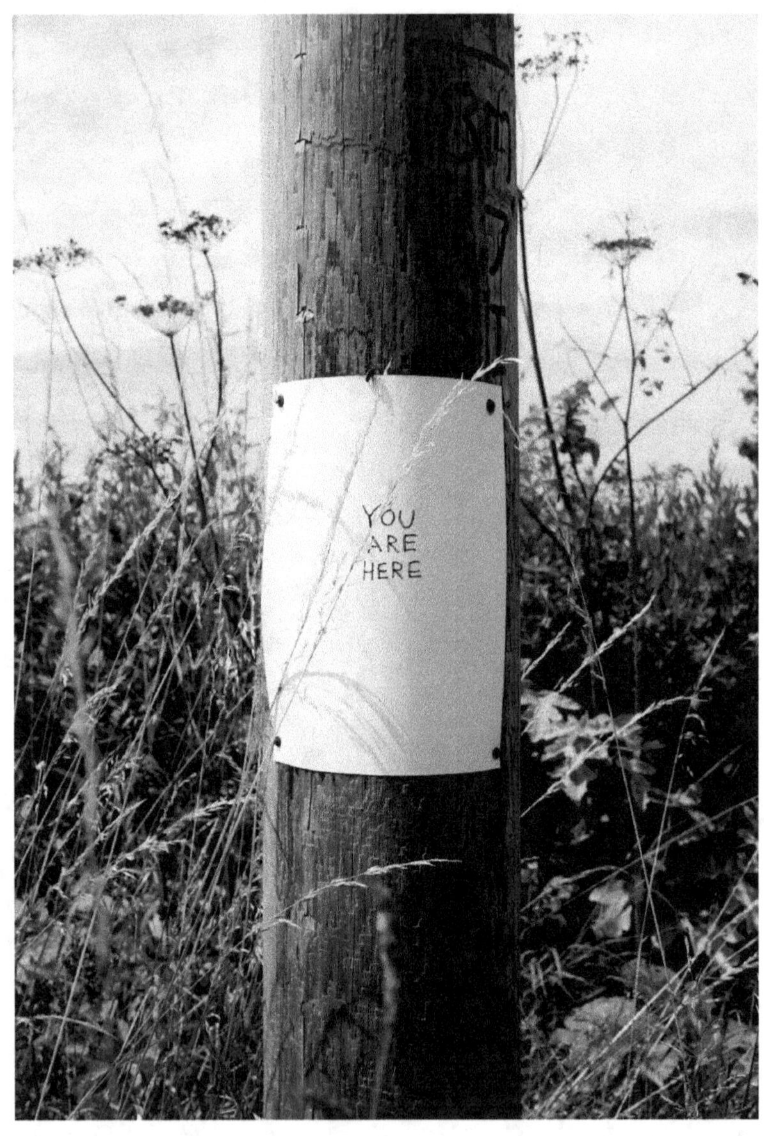
YOU
ARE
HERE

Welcome to your guide to fitness over 50. You may be asking yourself, can I be fit at my age? The simple answer is yes!

Whether you've been an athlete your entire life, were an athlete in your younger years or have never done anything exercise related, you can be fit.

Let's start by defining what is meant by the word "fit". For the purposes of this book, being fit is having a consistent focus on achieving health, vitality, energy and a clear mind. Being fit is improving your overall health through diet and exercise, wherever you currently are in your fitness journey. You will hear a couple of concepts throughout this book; be consistent and listen to your body. These may be the most important on your fitness journey. So, with that basis, let's begin your journey to being fit over 50.

The purpose of this book is to encourage you to start living a fit life even if you have or encourage you to start now. This is not a comprehensive guide for bodybuilding, preparing for a marathon or even a complete workout plan. The purpose is simply to get you started and encourage you to make necessary lifestyle changes that will impact your life for the positive and to live a fit life in your 50's and beyond.

So, I encourage you to read on and start living a fit life for you, your family and all of those in your life now and into the future

1

Chapter 1

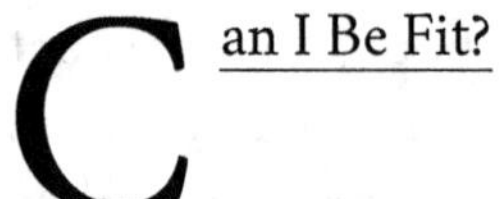

C an I Be Fit?

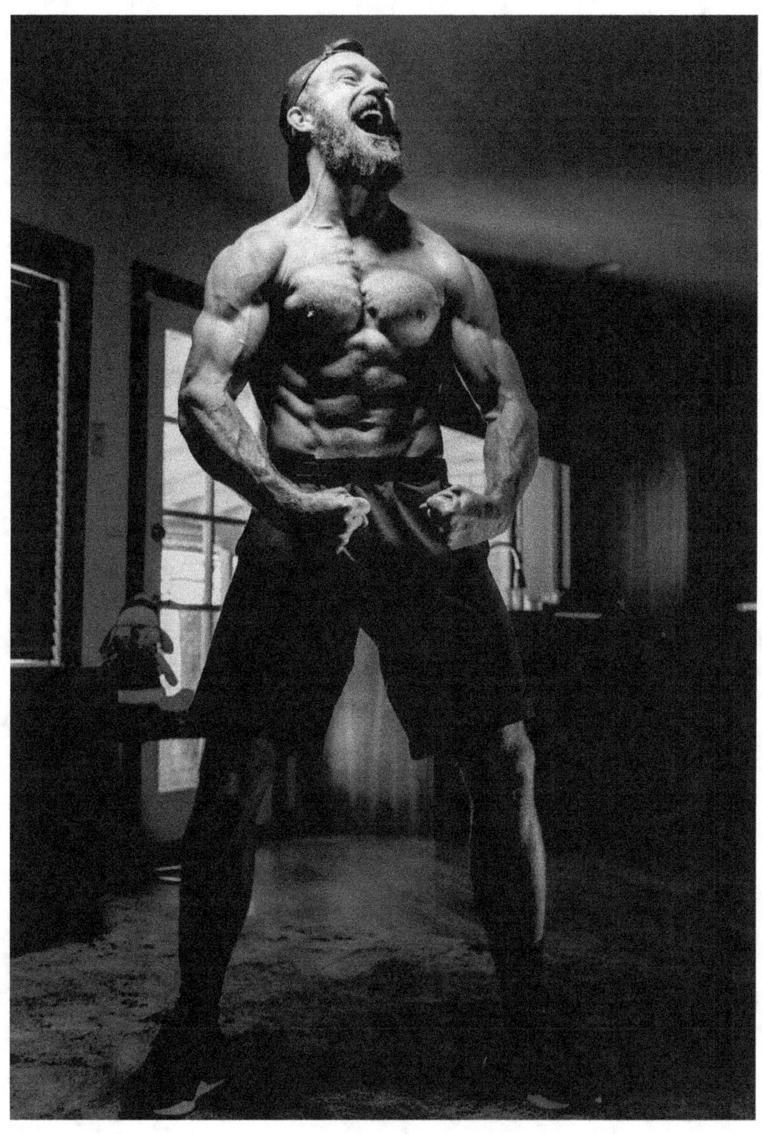

Being fit has many benefits to your overall health. Staying active, eating properly, keeping your mind active are all aspects of living healthy, vibrant and with energy. It's when we are not active that our body over time will start to deteriorate for lack of use. We've all heard the phrase, "use it or lose it", well this is what Im talking about. If you do not use your muscles and your connective tissues as they are designed to be used, you lose that ability. Feed with your mind, stay active,read books, learn new skills and read your Bible. These things contribute to your overall fitness and health.

If you have some health concerns, you should discuss with your physician and get their perspective on you starting any program. That being said, I believe that everyone can start some type of fitness program no matter the limitations.

To start a fitness program I would recommend a few basic "tests" to establish a baseline of where you are, even if you've never worked out in your life. An easy way to do this is to test three things, Cardio endurance , push-up strength test, and body composition.

Cardio endurance to give you a targeted heart rate and maximum heart rate. How many push-ups can you do in one minute (if you choose, you can do these on your knees but only if you have to)? And, measure your waist circumference. These are basic and will give you an idea of where you are physically.

If you're like me, you will need to warm up. Being a former athlete and playing football it takes me 5-10 minutes to get my body warm. I also have to start off slow until my body is completely warmed up. I do this by gently swinging my arms across my body, making small circles forward and backwards with my arms, some body squats and knees up.

Again, listen to your body and do what's comfortable. We are not setting any records here just getting warmed up.

1. For reference here is how to get our targeted heart rate…

Aerobic fitness: Target heart rate zone

The target heart rate zone is a heart rate range that gives your heart and lungs a good workout. This zone ranges from 50% to 85% of the maximum heart rate (MHR) for your age. Aim for 50% to 70% of MHR when you do moderately intense activities and 70% to 85% of MHR when you do vigorous activities.

You can use the target heart rate zone as a guide to see how hard you're exercising. It's okay if you don't reach your target zone. Any activity is good for your health. If you're on the lower end of your target heart rate zone, you can try to increase your effort little by little to get more from your workout.

If you exercise regularly, you can stop briefly to check your heart rate at times during an aerobic workout. If you don't exercise regularly, you can do a simple test by checking your heart rate after a brisk 10-minute walk.

Age Target heart rate zone: Beats per minute Maximum heart rate: Beats per minute

25 100-170 200
35 93-157 185
45 88-149 175
55 83-140 165
65 78-132 155

2) Muscular Endurance test….Push-up test….

Muscular strength and endurance: Push-up test

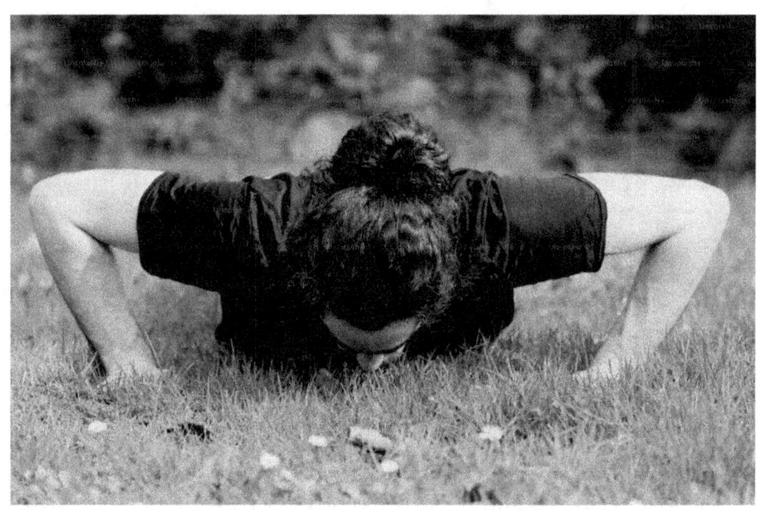

Measuring muscular fitness

Push-ups can help you measure muscular strength and endurance. If you're starting a fitness program, you can do push-ups on your knees. If you can, do regular push-ups. Follow these steps for both types:

- Lie face down on the floor with your elbows bent and your palms next to your shoulders.
- Keep your back straight. Push up with your arms until your arms are at full length.
- Lower your body until your chin touches the floor.
- Do as many push-ups as you can until you need to rest.

The following counts show a good fitness level based on age and sex. If your push-up count is below the target number, use the target as a goal to work toward. Counts above the targets mean better fitness.

Age Women: Number of push-ups Men: Number of push-ups

25 20 28

35 19 21

45 14 16

55 10 12

65 10 10

3) BODY COMPOSITION TEST

Body composition: Waist circumference

If the size of your waist, called the circumference, is greater than your hips, you carry more weight above the hips. This means you have a higher risk of heart disease and type 2 diabetes.

The risk is even greater for women with waist sizes of 35 inches (89 centimeters) or more. For men, the risk is higher with waist sizes of 40 inches (102 centimeters) or more.

With a cloth measuring tape, measure your waist just above the hip bones.

Body composition: Body mass index

BMI calculator

Your body mass index (BMI) shows whether you have a healthy amount of body fat.

You can find your BMI with a BMI table or online calculator.

To do the math yourself, divide your weight in pounds by your height in inches squared. Then multiply by 703. Or divide your weight in kilograms by your height in meters squared. To get your height in meters, divide your height in centimeters by 100.

The following shows what your BMI results mean.

BMI
Weight status
Below 18.5 Underweight
18.5-24.9 Normal weight
25.0-29 Overweight
30 and above Obese

These give you a base to help identify where you are on a fitness level. This is where you are today, so you will only improve from here.

A word on consistency….being consistent is one of the most important aspects of getting fit and maintaining a fit lifestyle. You should try to do something everyday. You may have planned a workout for the day and just aren't feeling it that day, that's fine. But do something…stretch, do deep breathing for 10 minutes, do 5 minutes of burpees or jumping jacks. Make sure you do something that day and then return to your planned workout the next day. Also, give yourself permission to take a day off. It's ok to skip a day, but make sure you get back to it the following day. Those days that you "force" a workout will many times be your best workout for the week. You will certainly feel great when you're finished and you conquered your goal for the day in your fitness journey.

In the next chapter we will discuss diet, and we will guide you in how to access your current dietary needs at present and what things to change.

2

Chapter 2

E ating Properly for Fitness

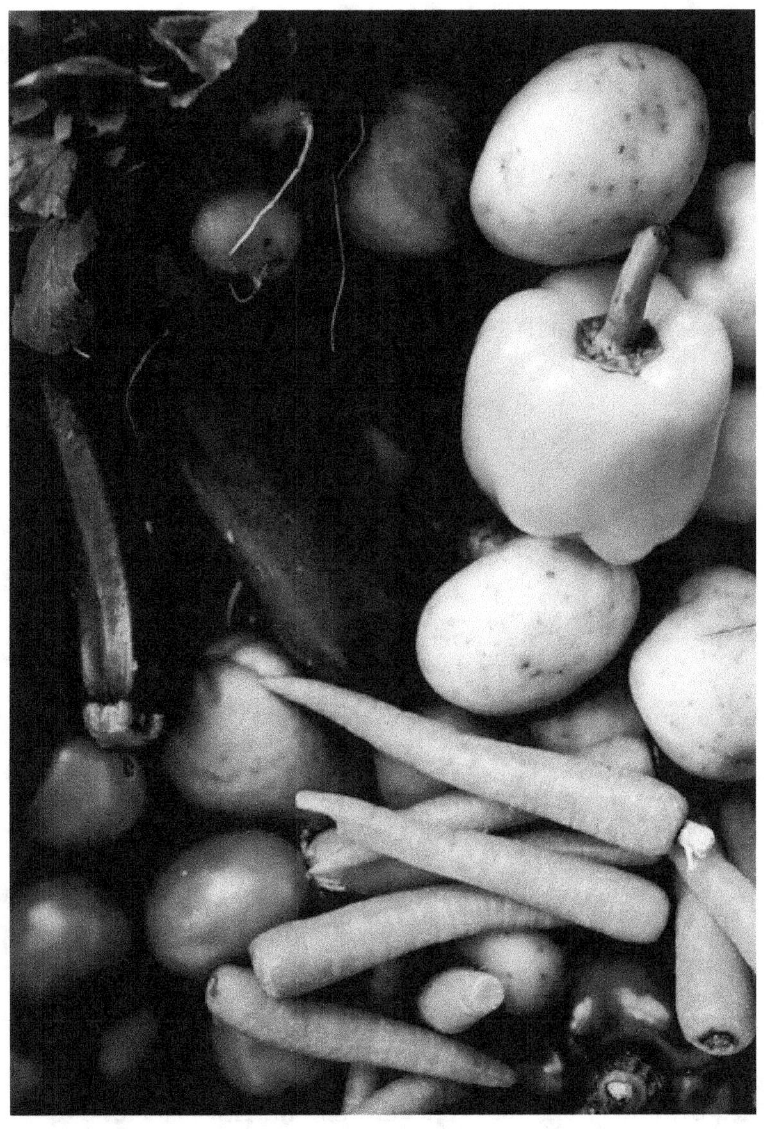

I submit that the most important aspect of being fit at any age is your dietary habits. You can eat anything and never see the results of your fitness goals. This may be the most difficult to maintain and habitual mentality to change.

Our bodies are designed to heal themselves given the proper nutrition and balanced diet. If we feed our bodies the proper nutrition, we will live daily with clear minds, energy, creativity and health.

The first step here is to track what you're eating on a daily basis. Get a notebook and write down everything you eat, drink and consume in a week. All the good and all the bad. Be honest with yourself; no one is watching or checking up on you. At the end of the day, you want a caloric deficit, not a surplus. You want to use all of the calories you consumed that day.

Once you have a record of a week's worth of eating, look up the caloric values of that food intake.

Here are some very general guidelines:
   If you want to weigh 150 lbs, you should eat no more than 1500 calories. If you want to weigh 200lbs, you should eat 2000 calories per day.

In my opinion, Your macronutrients should be 50% protein, 35% carbs, 15% fat. This works well for me and keeps me healthy and energetic and lean. Most nutritionists tend to be more carbs 50%, 30% protein and 20% fat. A mel sample with this in mind is provided at the end of this chapter. As always, listen to your body and play with the percentages that work for you. At the end of the day, it has to work for you. The key is to eat as clean and healthy as you can, choosing healthy fats over hardful fats, clean meats over processed meats and more complex carbs over simple surgery carbs. And allow a little cheating now and then, it's ok.

Protein is the building block of muscle and proper musculature, tendon and connective tissues. Proton is the second source of energy that your body uses. Protein sources are whole meats, chicken, beef, fish, venison, and some pork (though these are not the best). If you want to be leaner, stay with chicken and fish. No processed meats! The nitrates and preservatives are cancer causing and are not healthy for our bodies.

I prefer to buy meat from local farmers who you know do not use chemicals and steroids in their livestock and only use natural organic feed.

Carbs are the fuel your body uses for energy. Carbs are the first thing to be burned as energy. Of importance is that you're getting natural complex and simple cards. I would say more complex carbs. Desserts, cookies, cakes, candy and junk food are not considered carbs. Anything from a box is not whole foods.

Fats are very important to your overall health. Research now is pointing to the cause of many diseases from the lack of fat. Your brain operates on fat and research now tells us that the lack of fat causes dementia and Alzheimer's disease. That being said, you want healthy fats like Omega 3,6 and 9 oils. You get these from avocados, olive oil, nuts, coconut oil, fish such as salmon, olives. Again, stay away from processed foods and surgery desserts. These fats are toxic to your body and lead to long term health issues such as diabetes, high cholesterol and heart conditions.

Again, you don't have to go crazy with your eating habits. Sometimes you want a pizza or ice cream, I certainly do....You do not want this to be the norm but the exception. Moderation is fine. And being consistent with your eating habits, eating clean food and staying active are the most important points to be fit over 50.

Healthy Aging Foods to Focus On

- Fish (salmon and tuna, fresh or canned, halibut, haddock, cod and more)
- Shellfish (such as clams, mussels, oysters, shrimp)
- Nuts and seeds (including natural peanut butter and other nut or seed butters)
- Avocado
- Leafy greens
- Berries
- Eggs (eat the yolk!)
- Dark chocolate
- Pomegranate
- Fermented dairy (yogurt, kefir)
- Milk (dairy or fortified soy milk)
- Cruciferous veggies (broccoli, Brussels sprouts, cauliflower, cabbage)
- Coffee and tea

- Bone broth
- Oranges and other citrus fruits
- Carrots
- Beans (including canned) and lentils

Sample Clean Diet

- Prepare grilled chicken mixed greens salad with grated parmesan cheese to have for lunch on Days 2 through 5.

Day 1

Breakfast (317 calories)

- 1 serving omelet
- 1 cup blackberries, or blueberries

A.M. Snack (206 calories)

- ¼ cup roasted unsalted almonds

Lunch (345 calories)

- 1 serving 3 bean salad

P.M. Snack (110 calories)

- 1 cup low-fat mozzarella cheese stick

Dinner (533 calories)

- 1 serving Pan grilled salmon with olive oil
- ¾ cup cooked brown rice

Daily Totals: 1,511 calories, 78g fat, 87g protein, 116g carbohydrate, 30g fiber, 1,032mg sodium
   To make it 2,000 calories by adding a whey protein smoothie with blueberries and spinach for breakfast, plus add ¼ mixed mix nuts the P.M. snack.

Day 2

Breakfast (342 calories)

- 1 serving whey protein, Strawberry ½ banana smoothie

A.M. Snack (62 calories)

- 1 medium orange or apple

Lunch (445 calories)

- 1 serving grilled chicken mixed greens salad with grated parmesan cheese.
-
- ½ cup of black berries

P.M. Snack (115 calories)

- ½ cup low-fat plain Greek yogurt
- ½ cup raspberries

Dinner (514 calories)

- 1 serving chicken penne pasta with grilled asparagus with Italian seasoning and Olive oil
- *Daily Totals: 1,477 calories, 49g fat, 86g protein, 183g carbohydrate, 33g fiber, 1,360mg sodium*

To make it 2,000 calories: Add 1 serving Keto bread with Almond Butter and honey with half banana to breakfast to the A.M. snack and add 30 roasted unsalted almonds to afternoon snack

<u>Day 3</u>

Breakfast (337 calories)

- whey protein, Strawberry ½ banana smoothie

A.M. Snack (131 calories)

- 1 large apples

Lunch (445 calories)

- 1 serving grilled chicken mixed greens salad with grated parmesan cheese.
-

- ½ cup red grapes

P.M. Snack (131 calories)

- 10 dried walnut halves

Dinner (451 calories)

- 1 serving vegan lentil soup
-
- *Daily Totals: 1,495 calories, 56g fat, 84g protein, 179g carbohy-drate, 31g fiber, 1,123mg sodium*

To make it 2,000 calories: Add 32 dry-roasted unsalted almonds to the A.M. snack, plus add 1 serving guacamole salad to dinner.

Day 4

Breakfast (342 calories)

- 1 serving whey protein, blueberries ½ banana smoothie

A.M. Snack (110 calories)

- 1 cup low-fat plain kefir

Lunch (445 calories)

- 1 serving grilled chicken mixed greens salad with grated Parmesan cheese.
-

- ½ cup red grapes

P.M. Snack (131 calories)

- 1 large pear

Dinner (458 calories)

- 1 serving Grilled salmon with vinaigrette dressing and parmesan cheese
- 1-oz. slice keto bread

Daily Totals: 1,485 calories, 40g fat, 69g protein, 219g carbohydrate, 34g fiber, 1,487mg sodium

To make it 2,000 calories: Add 1 serving keto bread with almond butter, ½ sliced banana with honey to breakfast and add 1/4 cup dry-roasted unsalted almonds to the A.M. snack.

Day 5

Breakfast (337 calories)

- 1 serving whey protein, Strawberry ½ banana smoothie

A.M. Snack (32 calories)

- ½ cup raspberries

Lunch (445 calories)

- 1 serving grilled chicken mixed greens salad with grated parmesan cheese.
-
- ½ cup red grapes

P.M. Snack (157 calories)

- 12 dried walnut halves

Dinner (516 calories)

- 1 serving Chicken Kale soup
- 1 serving Guacamole salad

Daily Totals: 1,487 calories, 78g fat, 91g protein, 119g carbohydrate, 30g fiber, 1,402mg sodium

To make it 2,000 calories: Add 1/4 cup dry-roasted unsalted almonds to the A.M. snack, increase to 20 dried walnut halves and add 1 medium apple to the P.M. snack, plus add a 1-oz. slice keto bread for dinner.

Day 6

Breakfast (342 calories)

- 1 serving whey protein, Strawberry ½ banana smoothie

A.M. Snack (231 calories)

- 30 dry-roasted unsalted almonds

Lunch (366 calories)

- 1 serving Chicken and Kale soup
- 1 medium apple

P.M. Snack (131 calories)

- 1 large pear

Dinner (406 calories)

- 1 serving Baked Salmon, steamed broccoli
-
- *Daily Totals: 1,477 calories, 48g fat, 75g protein, 202g carbohy-drate, 41g fiber, 1,293mg sodium*

To make it 2,000 calories: Add 1 serving Keto bread with almond butter, ½ sliced banana, honey sandwich to breakfast and add 18 dried walnut halves to the P.M. snack.

Day 7

Breakfast (317 calories)

- 1 serving Omelette With mushrooms and ⅛ cop of cheese
- 1/2 cup pineapple

A.M. Snack (206 calories)

- ¼ cup roasted unsalted almonds

Lunch (366 calories)

- 1 serving tuna salad with
- ½ avocado

P.M. Snack (110 calories)

- 1 cup yogurt ice cream

Dinner (506 calories)

- 1 serving Lean hamburger or salmon grilled
- 2 cups spinach
- 1 mozzarella stick

Daily Totals: 1,506 calories, 79g fat, 79g protein, 127g carbohydrate, 30g fiber, 1,702 mg sodium

To make it 2,000 calories: Add 1 serving of whey protein and blueberry smoothie breakfast, plus add 1 1/2 tablespoons natural peanut butter to the apple at lunch.

Fasting

Have you ever fasted? If you haven't, it probably sounds scary or intimidating. Think about how busy our body is breaking down all the food and toxins we take in every day … it's a lot. And if you haven't given our bodies the proper treatment and nutrients to do this daily work, it is having to work overtime.

Fasting gives your body a much needed break from all that work…research shows that fasting one day a month does our bodies so much good. Even better fasting one day a week or intermittent fasting really helps.

I encourage you to give it a try. The easiest is intermittent fasting because most of this is done while you're sleeping. Here's a sample of how to do it:

Stop eating at 8:00pm one evening, only drink water before bedtime. Sleep 8 hours through the night. When you wake up, drink 16oz of water but do not eat anything. Then at lunchtime, have a sensible meal. You just fasted 16 hours! This is also a way to lose weight by intermittent fasting everyday. Of course the key is to eat normal meals for lunch and dinner and then start again at 8:00pm. Just another suggestion for you to try out.

Chapter 3

Cardio–the dreaded

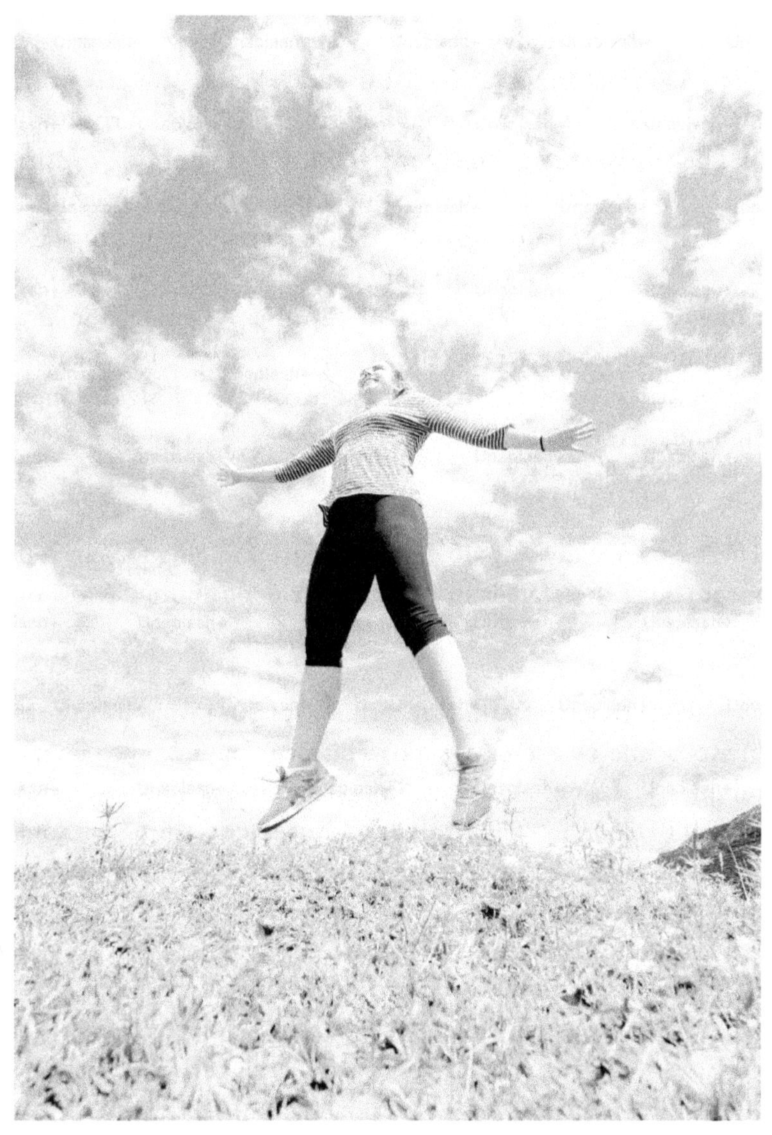

I am an old offensive lineman. Generally, I am a big guy. I've tried marathons and triathlons. The last time I ran a marathon my back prevented me from finishing. Turns out I had degenerative disk disease in and thinning of other disks in my lower back. I was in excruciating pain when I went in to see the Orthopedic physician. He told me that as a big guy I was made to push things not run. Every step I was taking while running was 750 pounds on my discs every step. So, my running career was over. After a year to recover, I started on a new fitness program that did not involve any long distance running.

HOORAY!!!

There are so many ways to get your heart pumping to help you meet your fitness goals that do not include running. Most of us say YES! Some of you, if you enjoy running, go for it...

My favorite types of cardio are walking for 30-45 minutes, short bursts of energy exercises such as burpees, mountain climbers, jumping jacks, punching bag, jump rope and box jumps. I also like HITT training which involves resistance training without stopping in your routine until you're finished; no breaks for 30 minutes straight.

Some like to ride a bike or a stationary bike. I like going on a bike ride but not for a long period of time. My dad who is 83 rides his stationary bike 4x/week for 20 miles each. He loves it; for me this is too boring.

I personally mix it up because I get bored and I hate cardio, so I have to change it up. What's important is that I get in 3-4 days per week of cardio. My wife prefers to walk, very fast I mind you, I cannot keep up with her long legs… but she's out there at least days a week walking at the park…

Consistency! Find out what you enjoy the most and make it work for you.

<u>Sample Cardio workout</u>

1. 4 rounds, 30 second break between each round

Burpees 10 reps
   Mountain Climbers 20 reps
   Jumping Jacks 20 reps
   Side Laterals-15 reps

or, Walk briskly for 20 minutes around the park.

or, Jump rope for 3 minutes 5 time intervals.

If this is too much, cut times in half. Do one and then in week two add another and so on. Do what you can do, don't go crazy, and slowly add time or repetitions as you get into better condition. Consistency is more important than your times or how many repetitions you do.

4

Chapter 4

R esistance Training
My most enjoyable day.

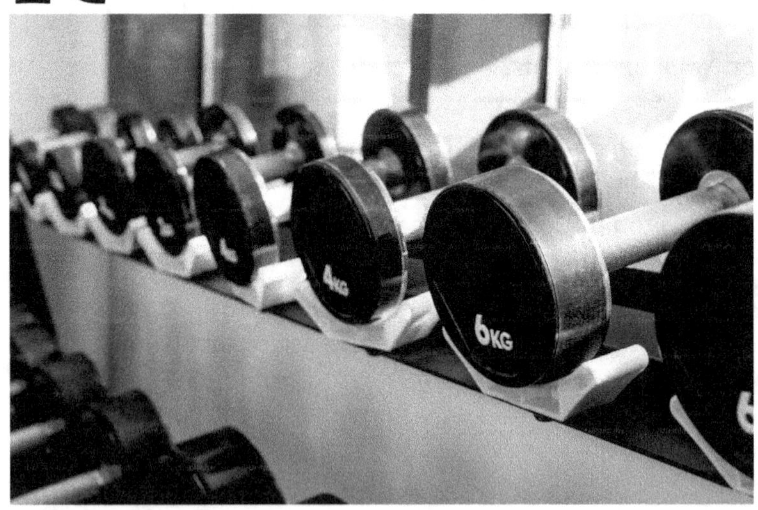

Resistance training is what I grew up doing for sports performance. As an athlete and football player you always wanted/needed to be stronger and faster. You train for your sport and the demands it puts on your body. As a football player who played offensive lineman, I needed to be explosively strong and be as big as I could get but still be able to move quickly.

Now I train a lot differently. My focus now is to stay active and healthy. I do not need to bench 400 pounds and run the 40 in 4.8. I just want to be fit and stay active as I get older.

Today in my resistance training I focus on the repetition range of 12-15 with as heavy of weight I can do for that repetition range. I use resistance bands, dumbbells, and kettlebells. Sometimes I do isometric exercises which are simply body weight exercises such as push-ups, sit-ups, dips and pull-ups.

I typically work different parts of my body each day. For example:
Monday Chest and Triceps
Tuesday Back and biceps
Wednesday Legs
Thursday Shoulders and Calves
I mix in abdominals and some cardio 3 times per week.

Sample weekly workout
Warm-up-10 minutes
Chest
Push-ups 3 sets of 12-15 repetitions
Dumbell presses 3x12-15 reps
Band chest flies 3x12-15 reps
Triceps

Push-downs 3x12-15 reps

Close-grip dumbbell press or diamond push-ups 3x12-15 reps

Overhead Tri Extension 3x12-15 reps

Abs

Heels to the Heavens 3x15 reps

Leg lifts 3x15 reps

Scissor leg lifts 3x15 reps

Stretch 10-15 minutes

Warm-up 10 minutes

Back DB rows 3x12-15 reps

Lat pull-downs with elastic band 3x12-15 reps

DB Deadlifts 3X12-15 res

Biceps/Forearms

DB Curls 3x12-15 reps

Concentration Curls 3x12-15 reps

Hammer Curls 3x12-15 reps

Stretch 10-15 minutes

Warm-up 10 minutes

Legs-quads, glutes, hams, calves

Air squats 3x25 reps

DB Squats 3x12-15 reps

Leg Curls 3x12-15 reps

Standing Calf Raises 3x12-15 reps

Stretch 10-15 minutes

Warm-up 10 minutes

Shoulders

Shoulder DB Press 3x12-15 reps

Side Lateral Raise 3x12-15 reps

Bent Over rear delt raise 3x12-15 reps

Abs

Crunches(dont pull on your head) 3x15 reps
Superman Arche 3x10 reps
Crunch side reaches 3x12 reps
Stretch 10-15 minutes

Isometric Sample Workout–no breaks between exercises.
Warm-up 10 minutes
Push-ups 3x15 reps
Bench dips 3x10 reps
Pull-ups 3x as many as you can, use assist if necessary
Leg raises 3x15 reps
Air Squats 3x20
Wall Sits hold for 30-60 seconds
Standing Calf raises 3x20

Do this workout 3x a week and you will be surprised what a great workout it is....

High Intensity Interval Training (HIIT)

HIIT Benefits

HIIT workouts are very effective. For many of the following fitness benefits, High-Intensity Interval Training is the best way to achieve them.

1. Burn a lot of calories in a short time.
2. High metabolic rate hours after exercising (which also helps increase overall).
3. Lose fat without losing muscle (can even gain muscle using HIIT while cutting weight if you eat a high protein diet).

4. Improves oxygen consumption and blood flow to muscles.
5. Reduces resting heart rate.
6. Reduces blood pressure (mainly for those who are over-weight).
7. Lowers blood sugar levels (great for people with type 2 diabetes).

You could mix in a HIIT plan into one of the days of your weekly workout.

If you are doing resistance training and cardio, your weekly plan can look like this:

- Day 1: Resistance Training
- Day 2: Cardio
- Day 3: HIIT
- Day 4: Rest
- Repeat

Or, you could work in two HIIT workouts into your weekly plan. Play with what you enjoy to help make a lasting lifestyle change.

Type of HIIT exercises:

-Burpees-Box Jumps

-Mountain Climbers-Sprints
  -Tuck Jumps-High Knees
  -Lateral Lunges with Hops
  HIIT workouts are explosive movements and this is key for an effective workout.
  HIIT exercises can be difficult so here is an example of durings for each

18 HIIT Exercises for Beginners:

  1. Tempo Squats (0:05)
  2. Lateral Squats (0:16)
  3. Squat to Inchworm (0:27)
  4. Up Downs, Low Impact (0:41)
  5. Up Downs, High Impact (0:55)
  6. Lateral Skiers, Low Impact (1:08)
  7. Lateral Skiers, High Impact (1:19)
  8. Shuffle | Reverse Lunge (1:30)
  9. Fast Feet (1:41)
  10. Elevated Push Up | Mountain Climbers (1:48)
  11. Butt Kicks (2:02)
  12. Lateral Shuffle (2:10)
  13. Bear Crawl (2:21)

14. Power Lunge (2:33)
15. High Knees (2:44)
16. Jumping Jacks (2:53)
17. Squat | Lateral Kick (3:04)
18. Jab | Cross | Shuffle (3:17)

Every exercise is to be at your own pace. If you're uncomfortable doing an exercise, stop. If you feel like your muscle is strained a little on one of the repetitions, stop. Do not injury yourself. Always listen to your body; it will tell you if you have gone too far. Also, use a weight that you can handle with proper form. Trying to go too heavy and cause injury will actually hinder your fitness goals. Start slow and with light weight until you use the proper range of motion and the weight becomes too easy. Then you can gradually add weight. Never sacrifice form over "muscling" up a weight; this only leads to injury. We are not trying to set any records…

That being said, you want to challenge yourself to push yourself and make sure you are getting the maximum out of your fitness program.

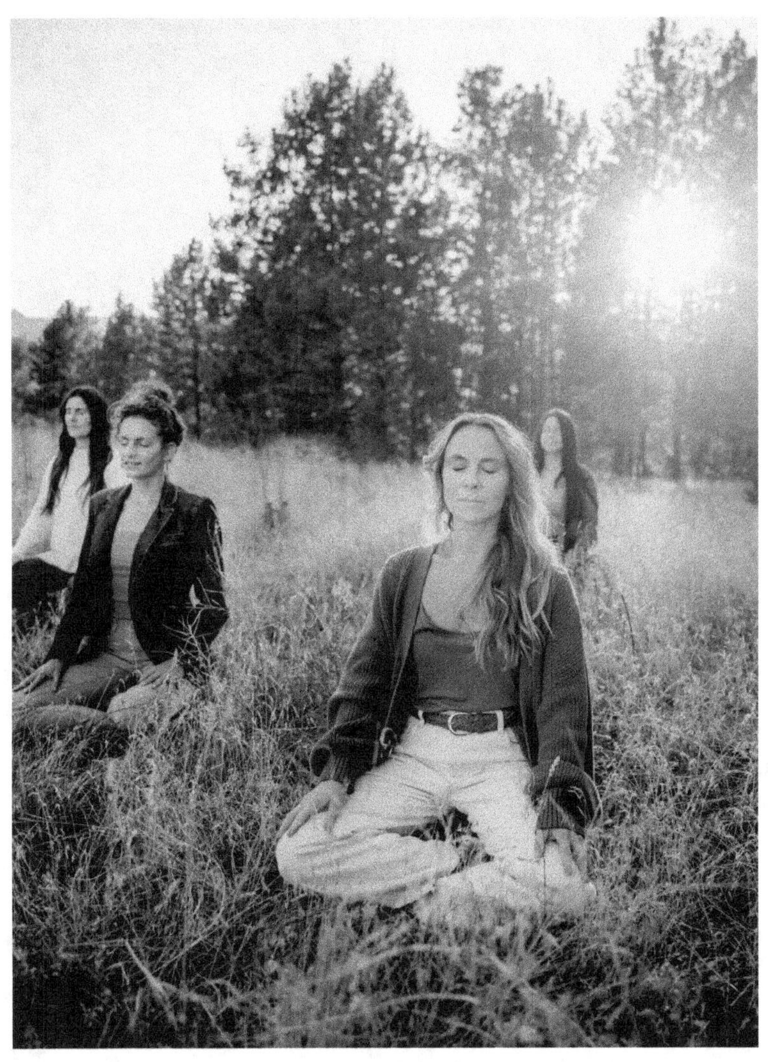

5

Chapter 5

I njury Prevention and Stretching

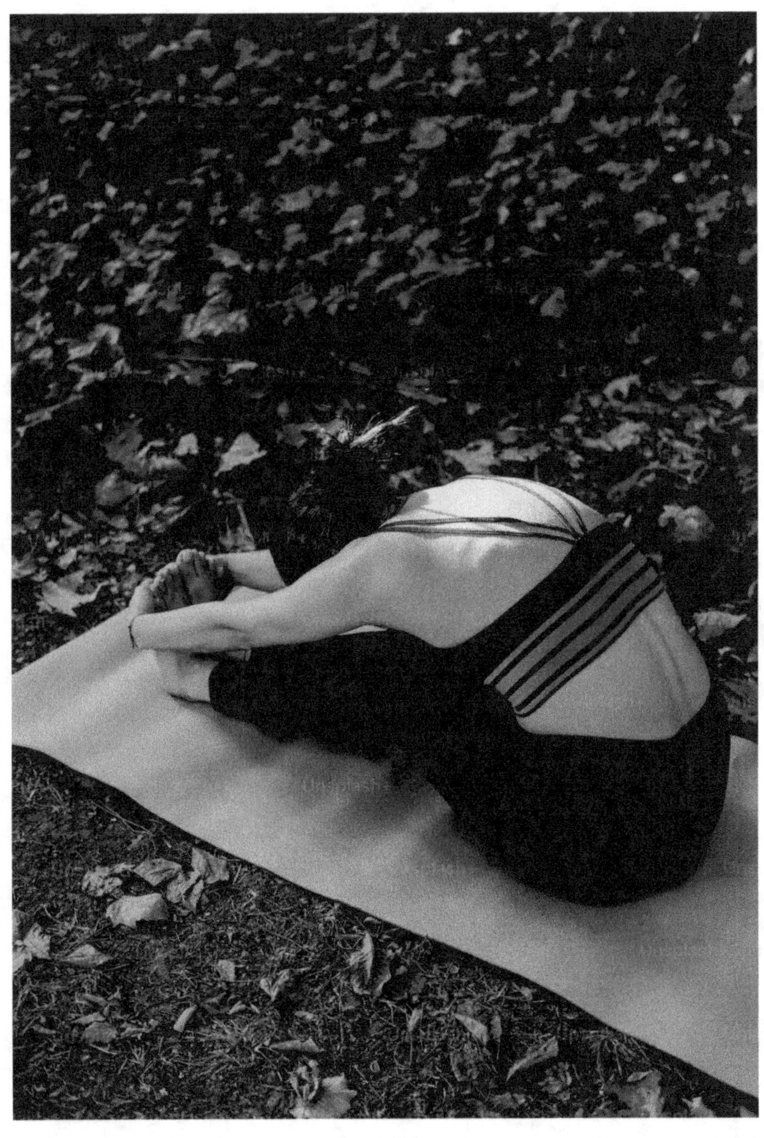

Injury prevention is most important as we get older and as we start any fitness program. If you perform the exercises properly as they are intended and use the correct resistance, you will prevent injuries. Proper form is paramount, using the weight that you can handle for your fitness level. If you are just starting out and have never done a fitness program, I could start with isometric only exercises, using your body weight as the resistance. You still must use the proper form and perform the exercise in the correct manner and in the range of motion it is designed to be completed.

If you're like me, it takes me at least 10 minutes to warm my body up…my shoulders, knees and back need extra time just to get ready to start any exercises. Doing this goes a long way to prevent injury; I've learned that the hard way.

In addition to that, stretching is a must but after your body is warm from your workout. You never want to stretch a cold muscle, so you always stretch at the end of your workout session. I've found that if I skip stretching, I will wake up with a sore stiff back. Not just sore but in pain. Everyone is different, and you must listen to your body, but stretching is vital to help with flexibility and injury prevention.

<u>Sample Stretching routine:</u>
   Standing hamstring stretch-stand, bend over with legs straight and just hang there for 30 seconds

Cross body arm/shoulder stretch. Reach across your body and gently push back of your arm to stretch your shoulders. Each shoulder for 30 seconds

Quad stretch, hold foot up behind your body stretching the front of your leg. Each leg for 30 seconds.

Neck rolls, roll your neck gently in all directions. Roll each side all around for 30 seconds.

Calf raise, step on a block or raised curb and let heel hang off, feel the stretching of each calf. Hold each calf for 30 seconds.

Lower back. Lay on the floor with your butt as close to the wall as possible and put your legs straight up the wall. Try to straighten your leg. Sit there for 3+ minutes.

Triceps raise your arm and bring it behind your head reaching as far down your neck as possible. Hold each arm there for 30 seconds.

Biceps and Forearms. Raise your arm with palm facing up, with the other hand gently push your fingers down stretching biceps and forearms. Hold each arm 30 seconds.

6

Conclusion

A<u>Call to Action</u>

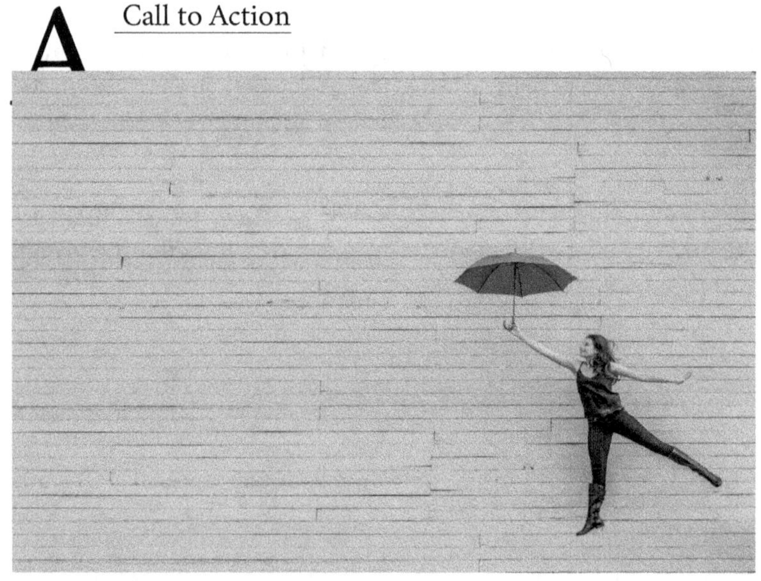

I want to encourage you to fiercely pursue your fitness every day. Do not let anything distract you from living fit and being as healthy as you can. Take a walk, do some resistance training, read your Bible, meditate, do deep breathing exercises, get outside and enjoy God's creation, laugh, enjoy friends and family. Tell the people in your life that you love them and how much they mean to you. Hug your spouse and your kids multiple times a day. A five second hug changes everything.

Dedicate yourself to loving wholly and fit and you will see that your life and others around you will be blessed.

You owe it to yourself and all the others in your life who you love and who love you.

So, now you have the basic knowledge to start your journey to being fit. Now you have to do the rest. This is book is only the beginning to help you get started. Do not be afraid to try different exercises, and rep ranges, eating different foods and different combinations of foods. I simply gave you small examples to help you start.

Also, if you do not like resistance training, that's fine, isometric exercises are very effective. Walking is very effective. The biggest part of all of this is eating better and start moving. As you get into your fitness journey you will probably try all sorts of different things, and that's perfectly fine. Find what you like and stick with it.

So, with that, I will say goodbye and here's to you living a more it life!

Blessings to you and all your loved ones.

Afterword

References

https://www.mayoclinic.org/healthy-lifestyle/fitness/in-depth/fitness/art-20046433 **"How fit are you? See how you measure up"**

https://www.eatingwell.com/article/7940188/meal-plan-for-healthy-aging-from-the-inside-out/
 "7-Day Meal Plan for Healthy Aging from the Inside-Out, Created by a Dietitian"

https://pmc.ncbi.nlm.nih.gov/articles/PMC8754590/
 Wang Y, Wu R. The Effect of Fasting on Human Metabolism and Psychological Health. Dis Markers. 2022 Jan 5;2022:5653739. doi: 10.1155/2022/5653739. PMID: 35035610; PMCID: PMC8754590.

https://www.setforset.com/blogs/news/hiit-for-beginners-best-exercises-workouts-tips
 "HIIT For Beginners: 18 Exercises, 5 Workouts & Tons of Training Tips"